What is Mental Health?

Mental health refers to cognitive, behavioral, and emotional well-being. It is all about how people think, feel, and behave. People sometimes use the term "mental health" to mean the absence of a mental disorder.

Mental health can affect daily living, relationships, and physical health.

However, this link also works in the other direction. Factors in people's lives, interpersonal connections, and physical factors can contribute to mental ill health.

Looking after mental health can preserve a person's ability to enjoy life. Doing this involves balancing life activities, responsibilities, and efforts to achieve psychological resilience.

Stress, depression, and anxiety can all affect mental health and disrupt a person's routine.

Although health professionals often use the term mental health, doctors recognize that many psychological disorders have physical roots.

WHO Responses

According to the World Health Organization (WHO) Trusted Source:

"Mental health is a state of mental well-being that enables people to cope with the stresses of life, realize their abilities, learn well and work well, and contribute to their community."

The WHO states that mental health is "more than just the absence of mental disorders or disabilities." Peak mental health is not only about managing active conditions but also looking after ongoing wellness and happiness.

It also emphasizes that preserving and restoring mental health is crucial individually and at a community and society level.

In the United States, the National Alliance on Mental Illness estimates that almost 1 in 5 adults experience mental health problems each year.

In 2020, an estimated 14.2 million adults trusted Sources in the U.S., or about 5.6%, had a serious psychological condition, according to the National Institute of Mental Health (NIMH).

All WHO Member States are committed to implementing the "Comprehensive mental health action plan 2013–2030", which aims to improve mental health by strengthening effective leadership and governance, providing comprehensive, integrated, and responsive community-based care, implementing promotion and prevention strategies, and strengthening information systems, evidence and research. In 2020, WHO's "Mental health atlas 2020" analysis of country performance against the action plan showed insufficient advances against the targets of the agreed action plan.

WHO's "World mental health report: transforming mental health for all" calls on all countries to accelerate the implementation of the action plan. It argues that all countries can achieve meaningful progress towards better mental health for their populations by focusing on three "paths to transformation":

> deepen the value given to mental health by individuals, communities, and governments; and match that value with commitment, engagement, and investment by all stakeholders, across all sectors;

- reshape the physical, social and economic characteristics of environments – in homes, schools, workplaces, and the wider community – to better protect mental health and prevent mental health conditions; and

- strengthen mental health care so that the full spectrum of mental health needs is met through a community-based network of accessible, affordable, and quality services and supports.

WHO gives particular emphasis to protecting and promoting human rights, empowering people with lived experience, and ensuring a multisectoral and multistakeholder approach.

WHO continues to work nationally and internationally – including in humanitarian settings – to provide governments and partners with the strategic

leadership, evidence, tools, and technical support to strengthen a collective response to mental health and enable a transformation towards better mental health for all.

Can your mental health change over time?

Can your mental health change over time? Yes, it's important to remember that a person's mental health can change over time, depending on many factors. When the demands placed on a person exceed their resources and coping abilities, their mental health could be impacted.

Over time, your mental health can change. For example, you may be dealing with a difficult situation, such as trying to manage a chronic illness, taking care of an ill relative, or facing money problems. The situation may wear you out and overwhelm your ability to cope with it. This can worsen your mental health. On the other hand, getting therapy may improve your mental health.

We all experience change. Change is fluid and can be negative or positive. When things change in your life, it can impact your mental health and well-being. You may even feel out of control in situations that you didn't expect. However, learning to manage the way you deal with these different situations will benefit your mental health.

When a good or bad change happens in your life, you'll need to adjust. Using healthy adjustment methods will help prevent negative effects on your mental health.

Why is mental health important for overall health?

Whether young or old, the importance of mental health for total well-being cannot be overstated. When psychological wellness is affected, it can cause negative behaviors that may not only affect personal health but can also compromise relationships with others.

Below are some of the benefits of good mental health.

1. A Stronger Ability to Cope With Life's Stressors

When mental and emotional states are at peak

levels, the challenges of life can be easier to overcome.

Where alcohol/drugs, isolation, tantrums, or fighting may have been adopted to manage relationship disputes, financial woes, work challenges, and other life issues—a stable mental state can encourage healthier coping mechanisms.

2. A Positive Self-Image

Mental health greatly correlates with personal feelings about oneself. Overall mental wellness plays a part in your self-esteem. Confidence can often be a good indicator of a healthy mental state.

A person whose mental health is flourishing is more likely to focus on the good in themselves. They will hone in on these qualities, and will generally have ambitions that strive for a healthy, happy life.

3. Healthier Relationships

If your mental health is in good standing, you might

be more capable of providing your friends and family

with quality time, affection, and support. When you're not in emotional distress, it can be easier to show up and support the people you care about.

4. Better Productivity

Dealing with depression or other mental health disorders can impact your productivity levels. If you feel mentally strong, it's more likely that you will be able to work more efficiently and provide higher quality work.

5. Higher Quality of Life

When mental well-being thrives, your quality of life may improve. This can give room for greater participation in community building. For example, you may begin volunteering in soup kitchens, at food drives, in shelters, etc.

You might also pick up new hobbies, make new acquaintances, and travel to new cities.

Types of mental health disorders

Specific mental disorders are grouped due to the features they have in common. Some types of mental illness are as follows:

- anxiety disorders

- mood disorders

- schizophrenia disorders

Anxiety disorders

According to the Anxiety and Depression of America, anxiety disorders are the most common mental illness.

People with these conditions have severe fear or anxiety related to certain objects or situations. Most people with an anxiety disorder try to avoid exposure to whatever triggers their anxiety.

Below are some examples of anxiety disorders.

1. Generalized anxiety disorder

Generalized anxiety disorder (GAD) involves excessive worry or fear that disrupts everyday living.

People may also experience physical symptoms, including:

- restlessness

- fatigue

- poor concentration

- tense muscles

- interrupted sleep

A bout of anxiety symptoms does not necessarily need a specific trigger in people with GAD.

They may experience excessive anxiety when encountering everyday situations that do not pose a direct danger, such as chores or appointments. A person with GAD may sometimes feel anxiety with no trigger at all.

2. Panic disorder

People with a panic disorder experience regular panic attacks involving sudden, overwhelming terror or a sense of imminent disaster and death.

3. Phobias

There are different types of phobia:

i. Simple phobias: These may involve a disproportionate fear of specific objects, scenarios, or animals. A fear of spiders is a typical example.

ii. Social phobia: Sometimes known as social anxiety, this is a fear of being subject to the judgment of others. People with social phobia often restrict their exposure to social environments.

iii.   Agoraphobia: This term refers to a fear of situations where getting away may be difficult, such as being in an elevator or a moving train. Many people misunderstand this phobia as the fear of being outside.

Phobias are deeply personal, and doctors do not know every type. There could be thousands of phobias, and what may seem unusual to one person can be a severe problem that dominates daily life for another.

4. OCD

People with obsessive-compulsive disorder (OCD) have obsessions and compulsions. In other words, they experience constant, stressful thoughts and a powerful urge to perform repetitive acts, such as handwashing.

5. PTSD

PTSD can occur after a person experiences or witnesses an intensely stressful or traumatic event.

During this type of event, the person thinks that their life or other people's lives are in danger. They may feel afraid or that they have no control over what is happening.

These sensations of trauma and fear may then contribute to PTSD.

Mood disorders

People may also refer to mood disorders as affective disorders or depressive disorders.

People with these conditions have significant mood changes, generally involving either mania, a period of high energy and joy, or depression. Examples of mood disorders include:

i. Major depression: An individual with major depression experiences a constant low mood and loses interest in activities and events that they previously enjoyed (anhedonia). They can feel prolonged periods of sadness or extreme sadness.

i. Bipolar disorder: A person with bipolar disorder experiences unusual changes in their mood, energy levels, levels of activity, and ability to continue with daily life. Periods of high mood are known as manic phases, while depressive phases bring on low mood.

ii. Seasonal affective disorder (SAD): Reduced daylight during the fall, winter, and early spring months trigger this type of major depression. It is most common in countries far from the equator.

Schizophrenia disorders

The term schizophrenia often refers to a spectrum of disorders characterized by psychotic features and other severe symptoms. These are highly complex conditions.

According to the NIMH, signs of schizophrenia typically develop between the ages of 16 and 30. The individual will have thoughts that appear fragmented and may also find it hard to process information.

Schizophrenia has negative and positive symptoms. Positive symptoms include delusions, thought disorders, and hallucinations, while withdrawal, lack of motivation, and a flat or inappropriate mood are examples of negative symptoms.

Risk Factors for Poor Mental Health

Your mental health is an important part of your well-being. This aspect of your welfare determines how you're able to operate psychologically, emotionally, and socially among others.

Considering how much of a role your mental health plays in each aspect of your life, it's important to guard and improve psychological wellness using appropriate measures.

Because different circumstances can affect your mental health, we'll be highlighting risk factors and signs that may indicate mental distress. But most importantly, we'll dive into all of the benefits of having your mental health in its best shape.

Mental health is described as a state of well-being where a person is able to cope with the normal stresses of life. This state permits productive work output and allows for meaningful contributions to society.

However, different circumstances exist that may affect the ability to handle life's curveballs. These factors may also disrupt daily activities, and the capacity to manage these changes.

The following factors, listed below, may affect mental well-being and could increase the risk of developing psychological disorders.

1. Childhood Abuse

When a child is subjected to physical assault, sexual violence, emotional abuse, or neglect while growing up, it can lead to severe mental and emotional distress.

Abuse increases the risk of developing mental disorders like depression, anxiety, post-traumatic stress disorder, or personality disorders.

Children who have been abused may eventually deal with alcohol and substance use issues. But beyond mental health challenges, child abuse may also lead to medical complications such as diabetes, stroke, and other forms of heart disease.

2. The Environment

A strong contributor to mental well-being is the state of a person's usual environment. Adverse environmental circumstances can cause negative effects on psychological wellness.

For instance, weather conditions may influence an increase in suicide cases. Likewise, experiencing natural disasters firsthand can increase the chances of developing PTSD. In certain cases, air pollution may produce negative effects on depression symptoms.

In contrast, living in a positive social environment can provide protection against mental challenges.

3. Biology

Your biological makeup could determine the state of your well-being. A number of mental health disorders have been found to run in families and may be passed down to members.

These include conditions such as autism, attention deficit hyperactivity disorder, bipolar disorder, depression, and schizophrenia.

4. Lifestyle

Your lifestyle can also impact your mental health. Smoking, a poor diet, alcohol consumption, substance use, and risky sexual behavior may cause psychological harm. These behaviors have been linked to depression.

Signs of Mental Health Problems

When mental health is compromised, it isn't always apparent to the individual or those around them. However, there are certain warning signs to look out for, that may signify negative changes for the well-being. These include:

- A switch in eating habits, whether over or interesting.

- A noticeable reduction in energy levels.

- Being more reclusive and shying away from others

- Feeling persistent despair

- Indulging in alcohol, tobacco, or other substances more than usual

- Experiencing unexplained confusion, anger, guilt, or worry

- Severe mood swings

- Picking fights with family and friends

- Hearing voices with no identifiable source

- Thinking of self-harm or causing harm to others

Diagnosis

Diagnosing a mental health disorder requires a multi-step process. A doctor may begin by looking at a person's medical history and performing a thorough physical exam to rule out physical conditions or issues that may be causing the symptoms.

No medical tests can diagnose mental disorders. However, doctors may order a series of laboratory tests such as imaging exams and bloodwork to screen for other possible underlying causes.

They will also do a psychological evaluation. This includes asking about a person's symptoms, experiences, and how these have impacted their lives. Sometimes, the doctor may ask a person to fill out mental health questionnaires to get an idea about a person's thoughts, feelings, and behavior patterns.

Most mental health specialists use the American Psychiatric Association's (APA) Diagnostic and Statistical Manual of Mental Disorders (DSM-5) to make a diagnosis. This manual contains descriptions and specific criteria to qualify for a diagnosis.

Treatment

There are various methods for managing mental health problems. Treatment is highly individual, and what works for one person may not work for another.

Some strategies or treatments are more successful in combination with others. A person with a chronic mental disorder may choose different options at various stages in their life.

The individual needs to work closely with a doctor who can help them identify their needs and provide suitable treatment.

Below are some treatment options for people with mental ill health.

1. Psychotherapy, or talking therapies

This type of treatment takes a psychological approach to treating mental illness. Cognitive behavioral therapy (CBT), exposure therapy, and dialectical behavior therapy are examples.

Psychiatrists, psychologists, psychotherapists, and some primary care physicians carry out this treatment.

It can help people understand the root of their mental illness and start to work on more healthful thought patterns that support everyday living and reduce the risk of isolation and self-harm.

2. Medication

Some people take prescribed medications, such as antidepressants, antipsychotics, and anxiolytic drugs.

Although these cannot cure mental disorders, some medications can improve symptoms and help a person resume social interaction and a routine while working on their mental health.

Some of these medications boost the body's absorption of feel-good chemicals, such as serotonin, from the brain. Other drugs either boost the overall levels of these chemicals or prevent their degradation or destruction.

3. Self-help

A person coping with mental health difficulties may need to change their lifestyle to facilitate wellness.

Such changes can include reducing alcohol intake, sleeping more, and eating a balanced, nutritious diet. People may need to take time away from work or resolve issues with personal relationships that may be causing damage to their mental health.

People with conditions such as anxiety or depressive disorder may benefit from relaxation techniques, which include deep breathing, meditation, and mindfulness.

Having a support network, whether via self-help groups or close friends and family, can also be essential to recovery from mental illness.

How to Maintain Mental Health and Well-Being

Because mental health is so important to general wellness, it's important that you take care of your mental health.

To keep mental health in shape, a few introductions to and changes to lifestyle practices may be required. These include:

- Taking up regular exercise
- Prioritizing rest and sleep on a daily basis
- Trying meditation
- Learning coping skills for life challenges
- Keeping in touch with loved ones
- Maintaining a positive outlook on life

Another proven way to improve and maintain mental well-being is through the guidance of a professional. Talk therapy can teach you healthier ways to interact with others and coping mechanisms to try during difficult times.

Some myths and facts about mental health

There are several commonly held beliefs and misconceptions about mental health. Here are some examples.

Myth: A person with a mental health condition has low intelligence.

Fact: Mental illnesses can affect anybody regardless of intelligence, income, or social status.

Myth: Teenagers do not have mental health issues. They just have mood swings due to their fluctuating hormones.

Fact: While it is true that teenagers often have mood swings, it does not mean that they cannot have mental health issues. Half of all mental health conditions begin by age 14.

Myth: People with mental health illnesses are dangerous, violent, and unpredictable.

Fact: Many people are quick to label people doing mass violence and crime as "mentally ill." However, crimes committed by people with serious mental health disorders only make up 5% of all violent crimes.

Myth: Psychiatric medications are harmful.

Fact: Mental illnesses, like other health conditions, are real illnesses. These medications may be necessary to help them function normally, ease their symptoms, and improve their quality of life. They are not harmful or an "excuse" for people to avoid dealing with their problems.

Myth: People with bipolar disorder are moody.

Fact: Bipolar cycles last from weeks to months and do not change as fast as people's moods often do.

Myth: A person with a mental health condition is weak. Such conditions would not affect strong people.

Fact: Having a mental health condition is beyond choice or willpower. Anyone can have a mental health condition.

Myth: Bad parenting causes adolescents to have mental health conditions.

Fact: Many adverse experiences and factors may influence a person's mental health and well-being. Adolescents' relationships with their parents and family are just one factor. A person raised in supportive and loving homes and those raised in homes maintained by caregivers who need mental support can experience mental health difficulties equally.

Myth: People with mental health needs cannot keep and perform well in a job.

Fact: People with mental health conditions can perform well in a jobTrusted Source, especially in a supportive workplace that supports and promotes mental health.

Outlook

While mental health disorders are common, they vary in severity. Most people can manage their symptoms and lead full lives with the proper treatment and access to support.

For others, recovery may not look like going back to their lives before the mental health disorder but learning new ways to cope and gaining more control over their lives.

The prevalence of mental disorders tends to peak in people ages 18–25Trusted Source, but drops significantly in people aged 50 and over.

Having a mental health problem, especially depression, is strongly associated with severe chronic health conditions such as diabetes, stroke, hypertension, cancer, and heart disease.

Summary

The term mental health refers to a person's cognitive, behavioral, and emotional well-being. It affects how people react to stressors, engage with others, and make choices.

According to the WHO peak mental health is more than just the absence of mental health problems. It is the ability to manage existing conditions and stressors while maintaining ongoing wellness and happiness.

Factors such as stress, depression, and anxiety can negatively affect mental health and disrupt a person's routine.